This book is based on real events, real emotions and real conversations...

Dedicated to the students impacted by The COVID Pandemic of 2020...

March 19, 2020

Spring Break is over and I just found out I cannot go back to school yet. It has been 55 days since our state was first exposed to this deadly virus they are calling COVID19. This means the virus is only getting worse and I am beginning to worry now. So many people have lost their lives already and that scares me. What scares me more is that the schools have closed... what does that even mean? We just stop learning until this thing ends? What if it doesn't end... ever?

2

March 20, 2020 Day 56

So the plan is to still do school, just not AT school... we have to pick up packets of work each week and the school is giving us computers so we can video chat with our teachers for help with our work. I hope this is only a temporary, very temporary thing. Okay well I need to clean my room before anyone sees it in the background.

March 23, 2020   Day 59

    Today would have the been our first day back to school after Spring Break. Instead we get to go pick up computers from the school drive up station. Tomorrow we are supposed to use some video chat program called Zoom to pretend like we are in class. I am being dead serious.. this seems crazy.

March 24, 2020   Day 60

Today was lame, I actually got excited about the
dumb zoom meeting because I realized I would see
my friends... and I miss my friends. The problem
was, there were only 4 other kids that showed up and
none of us knew how to really do anything on zoom...
not even our teacher. Maybe I will skip it tomorrow.

April 1 2020   Day 68

I am so confused. First we thought only old people
died from the virus. I did not understand why I could
not go anywhere if could not get really sick anyway. I
thought it was dumb. Today that changed though. My
friend's cousin is in the hospital right now and not
doing very good. She is only 16 and is really sick
from the virus. what does this even mean for us now?

April 15, 2020   Day 82

Things are changing everyday and to be honest, I am scared. This virus is killing people.. not just older people. Babies have died, kids and teenagers have died too. My school called yesterday because I have not been getting all my work done...... REALLY! How am I supposed to care about review work when I could die tomorrow???

April 16, 2020   Day 69

Today I talked to my teacher. I feel so lost these days. Being stuck at home 24-7 sucks! I actually enjoyed talking to my teacher.. something is wrong with me. She said school right now could be a good distraction from the worry I am filled with. She is right I think. I need something else to do or I might drive myself crazy. We also found out that schools are going to be closed the rest of this school year. This virus is not going away and it is only getting worse every day.

May ?? 2020

I don't know what the date is today... it is hard to keep track when I never leave my house. My mom leaves once a week to go get food and stuff. The toilet paper is gone EVERYWHERE she says. I thought she was joking at first, but she was being serious. I am sorry but that is ridiculous. Toilet paper... why? If the world is going to end, Toilet Paper is the last item on my priority list. There are plenty of other options there... people are so dumb. This school year is almost over although I think it actually ended back in March.

May 25, 2020

So we have about one week left of school. I never
thought I would say this.. but I miss school. I miss my
friends and I even miss having a teacher in real life. The
world is going crazy right now and I don't even have
anyone to talk about it. I don't have someone to keep
me from going crazy with the rest of the world. Everyone
is so stressed out all the time.. will this ever end?

May 27, 2020

I heard the school is doing a drive through graduation
for the 8th grade students. How lame is that going to
be? I will go though because my cousin is in 8th grade
and he lives with us. I wonder if any of my friends
will be there. Not like I will see them since we will all
be stuck inside our cars!

June 3, 2020   Day 129

Okay so the graduation was actually kind of awesome.
When we first arrived in the drive through line there was
a table with a bunch of bags on it. There were also a
handful of teachers standing at that table. They handed
a bag to each 8th grade student in the cars. The bag had
some school swag in it. A few seconds later we were
handed another thing from another group of teachers.
This time it was my cousins awards. Right after that
table we drove under a giant balloon ceiling. There were
like 500 balloons zigzagged above the drive through. It was
so cool. At the end of the balloons, all the teachers from
the middle school were standing there with signs and
stuff.

I got to see all of my teachers. Every single teacher
and aide were standing there cheering. Except the
teachers handing out things at the tables. At the end of
the teachers the principal and vice principal were standing
and having the cars stop. The 8th grade student then got
out of the car and walked down a long sidewalk to get
their diploma and take a picture. The school board and
superintendent were standing on the sidewalk the cheer
the 8th grader on. Another teacher was standing with a
microphone and would say the 8th graders name as they
walked down the sidewalk. Then we pulled into the parking
lot and my cousin walked back to the car. It was not
lame like I thought.

July 5, 2020

Forth of July was boring. We are still not allowed to go around other people. More people are dying from the virus than ever before and now there is some new symptom for kids and teens that is killing them too. I am bored, I am sad, and now I am scared! I don't want to die. I don't want to get sick. I am never leaving my room again!

July 17, 2020

we just found out that school is going to start next
year all online unless something changes. My 8th grade
year, my last year of middle school and I wont even
get to see my friends again! I don't even know how I
feel right now. I am angry I think. why don't people
listen and follow the rules? we are getting worse and
other countries are getting better... why... because
they are following the rules.

15

August 10, 2020

well I started school online today. IT was better than last year because everyone knew what to do this time. Also almost all the students showed up. I got to see my friends, but I did not get to talk to them. This is torture really. It is like showing a starving person a hamburger but then eating it right in front of them. This is going to be horrible!

August 21, 2020

I have no motivation to work. I don't care about my grades right now. I don't care about anything. Maybe the virus will not be that bad. If it never goes away I will never have a normal life anyway. If I get the virus then I am safe from it right? Can you get it more than once? I might have to find out. Sorry school, for homework today I will not be reading chapter 3, I will be doing research on the virus.

August 23, 2020

So I have spent the last 2 days trying to find answers. The only discovery I made is that NO_ONE knows anything about this virus. There are no websites that have the same information. Everyone says something different. I am even more confused now than I was before. Maybe focusing on school is easier than dealing with the rest of the world.

August 28, 2020

215... two hundred and fifteen days. That is how long it has been since the world shut down and life became what it is now... pointless. I heard someone on the tv say something about a new system in place to let people know how bad the virus is in that community. I am getting frustrated. A new system? What about a vaccine, or treatment.. why are people giving up fighting this thing and instead creating systems to live with it forever!

September 1, 2020

I did not want to wake up today. My back hurts and I have a headache. I got in trouble today for not having my camera on in class. I don't feel good, I looked like crap so I kept it off. I did all my work, answered questions and asked questions. She knew I was sitting there on the other side of the screen.. so what is the big deal? Her camera is always off when she is at her house teaching us. who gets her in trouble for that? I always liked school, but not so much today!

September 5, 2020   Day 223

Yesterday we found out my Dad was exposed to the virus at work. He was tested and we are waiting to find out the results. For now he is all alone in my parents bedroom with a mini fridge and microwave, staying away from the rest of us. He says he feels fine, but I can see the truth. He has looked tired the last couple of days and I noticed he was grabbing his head yesterday often, like he had a bad headache. I still have a headache too. My throat hurts now too. I find it harder each day to get up for 'fake' school. I wonder what would happen if I did not show up anymore...

october 14, 2020   Day 262

So much has happened the last few weeks, and yet
nothing has happened at all. My Dad was Positive for
COVID, and so the rest of us got tested and my Mom
was negative, my brother was negative... but I was
positive too. I was more scared than I have ever
been in my entire life. My Dad and I ended up in
quarantine together. I drug my twin mattress in his
room about 30 minutes after I found out I had it and
told him I did not want to be stuck in my room
knowing I was sick too. It is the weirdest thing... I
really enjoyed quarantine with my Dad.

22

we talked for hours one day. I could not even remember the last time I had an actual conversation with my dad that did not involve yelling. I forgot to take my journal and computer with me so I missed school for 3 weeks too. I told my dad how school felt fake.. and so unfair. He sat and listened to me complain and cry and did not interrupt me once. It felt so good to complain and have a fit out loud. I have not been able to see my friends in person in over 6 months, and this kind of complaining could not be done over a text message. I told my dad how I felt about everything and that sometimes it is like all the adults have forgotten we are going through this thing too.

He hugged me so tight and told me he was sorry. He apologized for not paying more attention to how I and my brother were feeling about all of this. He apologized for our teachers being so clueless to the pain they are causing us. Then he said something that I will never forget. He said, "There are always going to be unexpected challenges in our lives, whether it is an event like this virus, or a person who tries to bring you down, they have one thing in common, you or I, we have no control over them. We can only control how we deal with each challenge, how we rise above them, or how we crumble in their presence. Regardless of how we face them, we do it knowing our actions, our thoughts, our words, they are all in our control...

This Pandemic sucks, being sick sucks even more, but I do not worry about ways to change it, because I know I have no control over it. You have no control over the adults in your life, so do not let their poor choices, their selfish acts or cold words control you.

You have control of your reaction to them. Tell them, each and everyone of them, how they are making you feel. You will see how your controlled choices can influence change. Just because they do not seem to notice the struggle you are going through, does not mean they do not care."

I asked him why he thinks that... I thought he was just trying to make me feel better... but he answered my question like this, "Because I had no idea you were struggling to cope with all of this, I was not noticing how unhappy you were.. and I love you, I care about you and your brother more than anything else in this world. our conversations the last couple of days has opened my eyes to so many things..

If you tell your teachers how you feel and nothing changes, I will not make you continue attending the online class sessions.. we will figure something else out.

October 17, 2020

I keep thinking about what my Dad told me in quarantine. I have to focus on what I can control and not stress out about the rest. I have control of my mood, my words, my own actions. I am going to try something new tomorrow during my class session. My Dad told my mom everything and I have noticed her being more patient with us, but I see this sadness in her eyes now.

October 19, 2020

School has changed, I have decided to make the most of it. I ask questions all day. Even if I know the answer, or already understand what my teacher is explaining, I act like I am confused. This has made her teach us again. Really teach us. I can tell a few of the students are glad I am doing this. More students are showing up for class at the end of the day now, and my teacher has even added free time each period for us to just talk to our friends about whatever we want. I did not tell her everything, but I emailed her and told her about me and my Dad getting sick.

I also told her I realized how much I missed my friends, and how I had been holding in so many things because I did not have my friends to talk to. I asked her if there was anyway to allow us to use our breaks to stay in the class sessions and just talk to each other. She actually made time during our classes for it! My Dad was right and I feel so much better about everything now. Maybe I will survive this Pandemic after all.

Day 267